This Medication Book Belongs To:

____

If Found Call:

____

Emergency Contacts

Name	Phone #	Additional Information

Doctors Contact Information

Name	Phone Number

Doctors Contact Information

Name	Phone Number

Insurance Information

Company

____

Policy#

____

Group #

____

Phone #

____

Insurance Information

Company

____

Policy#

____

Group #

____

Phone #

____

Upcoming Appointments

Doctor	Date	Time	Notes

Upcoming Appointments

Doctor	Date	Time	Notes

Upcoming Appointments

Doctor	Date	Time	Notes

Medication

Date

MEDS	Dose	AM	NOON	PM	Bed
MEDS	Dose	AM	NOON	PM	Bed

Vitamin Supplements and Over the Counter Medications Notes

Product	Dose	AM	PM

Medication

Date

MEDS	Dose	AM	NOON	PM	Bed
MEDS	Dose	AM	NOON	PM	Bed

Vitamin Supplements and Over the Counter Medications Notes

Product	Dose	AM	PM

Medication

Date

MEDS	Dose	AM	NOON	PM	Bed
MEDS	Dose	AM	NOON	PM	Bed

Vitamin Supplements and Over the Counter Medications Notes

Product	Dose	AM	PM

Medication

Date

MEDS	Dose	AM	NOON	PM	Bed

Vitamin Supplements and Over the Counter Medications Notes

Product	Dose	AM	PM

Medication

Date

MEDS	Dose	AM	NOON	PM	Bed
MEDS	Dose	AM	NOON	PM	Bed

Vitamin Supplements and Over the Counter Medications Notes

Product	Dose	AM	PM

Medication

Date

MEDS	Dose	AM	NOON	PM	Bed

Vitamin Supplements and Over the Counter Medications Notes

Product	Dose	AM	PM

Medication

Date

MEDS	Dose	AM	NOON	PM	Bed

Vitamin Supplements and Over the Counter Medications Notes

Product	Dose	AM	PM

Medication

Date

MEDS	Dose	AM	NOON	PM	Bed
MEDS	Dose	AM	NOON	PM	Bed

Vitamin Supplements and Over the Counter Medications Notes

Product	Dose	AM	PM

Medication

Date

MEDS	Dose	AM	NOON	PM	Bed

MEDS	Dose	AM	NOON	PM	Bed

Vitamin Supplements and Over the Counter Medications Notes

Product	Dose	AM	PM

Medication

Date

MEDS	Dose	AM	NOON	PM	Bed
MEDS	Dose	AM	NOON	PM	Bed

Vitamin Supplements and Over the Counter Medications Notes

Product	Dose	AM	PM

Medication

Date

MEDS	Dose	AM	NOON	PM	Bed
MEDS	Dose	AM	NOON	PM	Bed

Vitamin Supplements and Over the Counter Medications Notes

Product	Dose	AM	PM

Medication

Date

MEDS	Dose	AM	NOON	PM	Bed
MEDS	Dose	AM	NOON	PM	Bed

Vitamin Supplements and Over the Counter Medications Notes

Product	Dose	AM	PM

Medication

Date

MEDS	Dose	AM	NOON	PM	Bed
MEDS	Dose	AM	NOON	PM	Bed

Vitamin Supplements and Over the Counter Medications Notes

Product	Dose	AM	PM

Medication

Date

MEDS	Dose	AM	NOON	PM	Bed

Vitamin Supplements and Over the Counter Medications Notes

Product	Dose	AM	PM

Medication

Date

MEDS	Dose	AM	NOON	PM	Bed
MEDS	Dose	AM	NOON	PM	Bed

Vitamin Supplements and Over the Counter Medications Notes

Product	Dose	AM	PM

Medication

MEDS	Dose	AM	NOON	PM	Bed
MEDS	Dose	AM	NOON	PM	Bed

Vitamin Supplements and Over the Counter Medications Notes

Product	Dose	AM	PM

Medication

Date

MEDS	Dose	AM	NOON	PM	Bed

MEDS	Dose	AM	NOON	PM	Bed

Vitamin Supplements and Over the Counter Medications Notes

Product	Dose	AM	PM

Medication

Date

MEDS	Dose	AM	NOON	PM	Bed
MEDS	Dose	AM	NOON	PM	Bed

Vitamin Supplements and Over the Counter Medications Notes

Product	Dose	AM	PM

Medication

Date

MEDS	Dose	AM	NOON	PM	Bed
MEDS	Dose	AM	NOON	PM	Bed

Vitamin Supplements and Over the Counter Medications Notes

Product	Dose	AM	PM

Medication

Date

MEDS	Dose	AM	NOON	PM	Bed
MEDS	Dose	AM	NOON	PM	Bed

Vitamin Supplements and Over the Counter Medications Notes

Product	Dose	AM	PM

Medication

Date

MEDS	Dose	AM	NOON	PM	Bed

Vitamin Supplements and Over the Counter Medications Notes

Product	Dose	AM	PM

Medication

Date

MEDS	Dose	AM	NOON	PM	Bed

Vitamin Supplements and Over the Counter Medications Notes

Product	Dose	AM	PM

Medication

Date

MEDS	Dose	AM	NOON	PM	Bed
MEDS	Dose	AM	NOON	PM	Bed

Vitamin Supplements and Over the Counter Medications Notes

Product	Dose	AM	PM

Medication

Date

MEDS	Dose	AM	NOON	PM	Bed
MEDS	Dose	AM	NOON	PM	Bed

Vitamin Supplements and Over the Counter Medications Notes

Product	Dose	AM	PM

Medication

Date

MEDS	Dose	AM	NOON	PM	Bed
MEDS	Dose	AM	NOON	PM	Bed

Vitamin Supplements and Over the Counter Medications Notes

Product	Dose	AM	PM

Medication

Date

MEDS	Dose	AM	NOON	PM	Bed
MEDS	Dose	AM	NOON	PM	Bed

Vitamin Supplements and Over the Counter Medications Notes

Product	Dose	AM	PM

Medication

Date

MEDS	Dose	AM	NOON	PM	Bed
MEDS	Dose	AM	NOON	PM	Bed

Vitamin Supplements and Over the Counter Medications Notes

Product	Dose	AM	PM

Medication

Date

MEDS	Dose	AM	NOON	PM	Bed
MEDS	Dose	AM	NOON	PM	Bed

Vitamin Supplements and Over the Counter Medications Notes

Product	Dose	AM	PM

Medication

Date

MEDS	Dose	AM	NOON	PM	Bed
MEDS	Dose	AM	NOON	PM	Bed

Vitamin Supplements and Over the Counter Medications Notes

Product	Dose	AM	PM

Medication

Date

MEDS	Dose	AM	NOON	PM	Bed

Vitamin Supplements and Over the Counter Medications Notes

Product	Dose	AM	PM

Medication

Date

MEDS	Dose	AM	NOON	PM	Bed
MEDS	Dose	AM	NOON	PM	Bed

Vitamin Supplements and Over the Counter Medications Notes

Product	Dose	AM	PM

Medication

Date

MEDS	Dose	AM	NOON	PM	Bed
MEDS	Dose	AM	NOON	PM	Bed

Vitamin Supplements and Over the Counter Medications Notes

Product	Dose	AM	PM

Medication

Date

MEDS	Dose	AM	NOON	PM	Bed
MEDS	Dose	AM	NOON	PM	Bed

Vitamin Supplements and Over the Counter Medications Notes

Product	Dose	AM	PM

Medication

Date

MEDS	Dose	AM	NOON	PM	Bed
MEDS	Dose	AM	NOON	PM	Bed

Vitamin Supplements and Over the Counter Medications Notes

Product	Dose	AM	PM

Medication

Date

MEDS	Dose	AM	NOON	PM	Bed
MEDS	Dose	AM	NOON	PM	Bed

Vitamin Supplements and Over the Counter Medications Notes

Product	Dose	AM	PM

Medication

Date

MEDS	Dose	AM	NOON	PM	Bed
MEDS	Dose	AM	NOON	PM	Bed

Vitamin Supplements and Over the Counter Medications Notes

Product	Dose	AM	PM

Medication

Date

MEDS	Dose	AM	NOON	PM	Bed

| MEDS | Dose | AM | NOON | PM | Bed |

Vitamin Supplements and Over the Counter Medications Notes

Product	Dose	AM	PM

Medication

Date

MEDS	Dose	AM	NOON	PM	Bed
MEDS	Dose	AM	NOON	PM	Bed

Vitamin Supplements and Over the Counter Medications Notes

Product	Dose	AM	PM

Medication

Date

MEDS	Dose	AM	NOON	PM	Bed

| MEDS | Dose | AM | NOON | PM | Bed |

Vitamin Supplements and Over the Counter Medications Notes

Product	Dose	AM	PM

Medication

Date

MEDS	Dose	AM	NOON	PM	Bed
MEDS	Dose	AM	NOON	PM	Bed

Vitamin Supplements and Over the Counter Medications Notes

Product	Dose	AM	PM

Medication

Date

MEDS	Dose	AM	NOON	PM	Bed

Vitamin Supplements and Over the Counter Medications Notes

Product	Dose	AM	PM

Medication

Date

MEDS	Dose	AM	NOON	PM	Bed

Vitamin Supplements and Over the Counter Medications Notes

Product	Dose	AM	PM

Notes

Notes

Notes

Notes

Notes

Notes

Notes